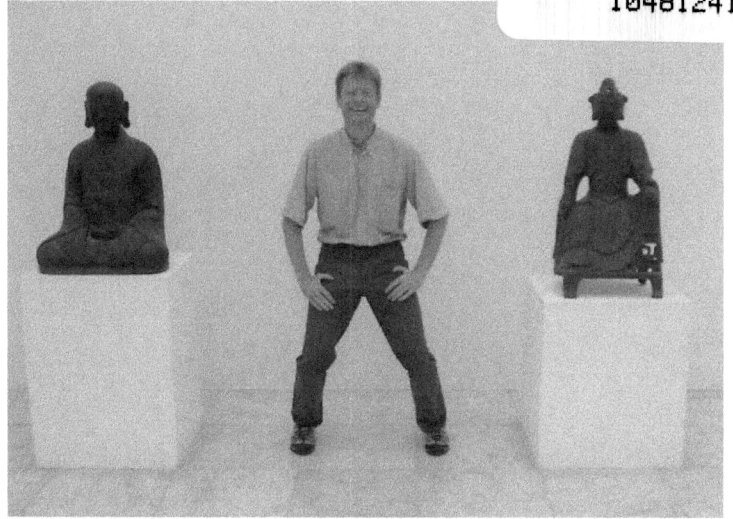

The Five Tibetans 2.0

Suitable for Late-Comers

by Dr. Stefan Ulrich Tippach Ph.D.

IMPRESSUM

Dr. Stefan U. Tippach Ph.D.

53121 Bonn

Endenicher Str. 287

Germany

www.Dr-Tippach.de

mail@Dr-Tippach.de

COPYRIGHT

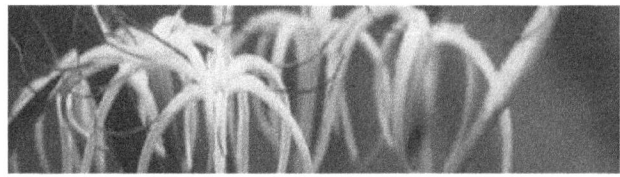

INVITATION

Learn with me the traditional exercises
called
"The Five Tibetan Rites"

It is a wonderful way to become and
stay healthy and well.

This book is for people with or without
prior knowledge, late-comers,
as well as ill and recovering people.

For those of you who know the Tibetans
well already, here is your chance
of going into depth!

Preface: Why this book is essential for your health

Tibet is an almost mystical word. "Five Tibetans" thus already has the air of a sort of "spiritual gymnastics". In some ways that is quite right, because the exercises you are going to learn are good for your body and your mental health. Overall, they will neatly serve your wellbeing in a physical way and equally in an emotional way. Even the West has understood by now that being well must include aspects of spiritual well-being. We have come far enough now to begin my version of the Tibetans 2.0.

The Tibetan Rites will certainly improve your joints and ligaments. Yet, far beyond that, they also harmonize energies in your body and help you maintain an overall balance. For instance, someone with a tense neck will learn to release the energy, which is blocked in this body part, and how to guide the "Qi" to the feet, where it is currently more needed. "Old stuff" is released, and we begin to build up newer, healthier components.

Some of the exercises have a reputation of being difficult. Some people, and in particular elderly people, think that they are incapable of performing these exercises. But relax! I have more than 20 years of experience training elderly persons who begun to exercise late in life. We call them late-comers. They can certainly also do it. In addition, I teach ill and recovering people. Hence, I made it my task to find ways of presenting the Tibetans in a modern 2.0 version, which is easy enough for everybody. For that to happen, I have inserted simplified versions and ways of doing an exercise in several steps until we tackle the entire exercise.

Moreover, I have added a complete explanation of the pauses and recovering phases between each exercise. It is of vital importance not to overstrain the body and give oneself always enough "Yin", i.e., softer and restful energies. This is in line with modern insights in breathing-, motion-, and gymnastics -therapy. You shall see and experience how your whole self is renewed.

In this book, I present help, correction and support for practically every age and condition. Everybody, and certainly not only latecomers, can profit immensely; for of course, I also show the entire exercise as well. One thing is for sure: we all need to move, especially when we are ill or older. Therefore, you will find in this book all Tibetans in their correct form and the steps leading up to them. He, who knows these steps will also know best how to coordinate their movement with their breathing. Hence, I can recommend my Tibetans 2.0 to the young and healthy as well!

Moreover, I teach mindfulness. I believe that before Yoga and Qi- Gong (cf. Tippach, Qi -Gong, "Opening the 9 Gates") took their separate ways, there was a much older tradition of exercising, which already contained astonishing insights into the functioning of the human body and mind. They knew about medical movement therapy and had anchored it in their exercises, part of which were the 5 Tibetans. This included the principle of mindfulness. Mindfulness allows us to avoid body positions or movements which our body cannot perform, or not right now, or not anymore. That makes it compelling to take my step-by-step approach, which I present herein. I offer everybody the opportunity to learn each exercise in stages, which are possible for all of you to perform. Improvements will may come a bit slower, but they will come to you. In the end, you will be able to slow down the rate at which you age, and eventually even reverse the process of aging. No external thing such as a facial cream can do that for you. Instead, invest some time in reading this and doing the exercises!

At the same time, you learn a small daily routine, which you can carry out every day without much effort or time. It is a marvellous contribution to your health and wellbeing. **Check out my videos and podcasts on healing and Qi-Gong! Support my work on**

www.patreon.com/user?u=14780777

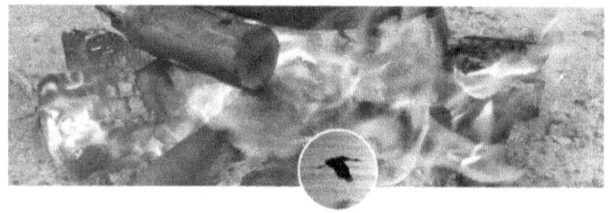

CONTENT OVERVIEW

Introduction

Basics for you Five Tibetans

Practice

Each of the Five Exercises

The Phases of Rest

Effects on your Health

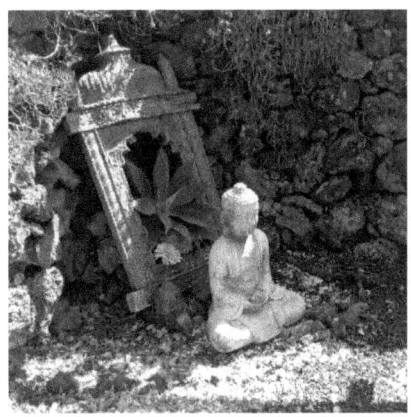

Thanking

My loving thanks goes to all my students and to the participants of my classes and workshops. It is due to your ques-
tions and interest that I was able to distill what is really
needed for exercising when we grow older and weaker. I also
thank you for your efforts and the smiles on your faces when
you became able to carry out the individual Tibetans.

I want to also thank everyone helping to create the book
along with the photos and videos, especially Benedikt Wieser
from Wieser Productions. Finally, I would like to thank Mrs.
Dorothee Rego Dacal for her inspired editing work.

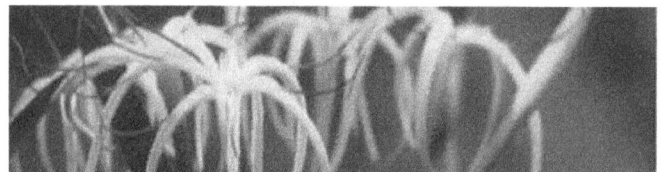

Contents

Introduction to the Five Tibetans 2.0

The exercises called "Tibetans", probably originate in Tibet or at least Tibetan territory. Especially in the westerns part of Tibet, we find many monasteries in which the monks not only practice spirituality, but also connect the physical with our spiritual existence. Maybe the exact place of origin will remain unknown, or maybe "Tibet" as a country or region has been added later on. There is enough evidence to accept that these exercises originate from the Himalayan region.

"Mind and Body" is a topic dating back to antiquity. The Romans had the saying "Mens sana in corpore sano", which many have heard in school. After all, it is in fact true: Spirit and body do not heal in separation, but only together. According to modern medicine, sports and exercising have a positive correlation to psychological diseases. For example, someone who is going through a phase of being depressed needs to stretch daily, at best several times. Stretching of the ligaments has a positive influence on our mood because it helps the body to produce serotonin. The Tibetan exercises contain several elements of stretching.

For anyone who doesn't like cold jumpstarting into exercise, I can recommend to warm up with my 12-Minutes-of-QiGong-programm (Opening the 9 Gates). After that sequence, the Tibetans can be exercised even more efficiently.

Carrying Out the Five Tibetans *Correctly*

When I say carry the 5 Tibetans out "correctly" I mean put them in the right context and get the moves right. This is because only then will one benefit from them in a health-promoting way. For us to do that, a certain flexibility is required. Participants in my workshops feel the same exact way. Indeed, at the beginning, some of the positions and moves seem to be quite an obstacle. Then, people watch some of my videos (PATREON) and think they "could never do that (again)". But that is far from the truth!

The exercises presented in this book (and in the related videos) are especially relevant to late-comers, people in recovery, and to elderly or ill people. That is because these exercises will help you gain your physical health back, along with your flexibility. What was missing up until now is a presentation which really takes the difficulties of age or illness into account. This small book closes the lamentable gap. I am going to describe the exercises from the very basics. Thus, everybody can move on step by step and improve their health gradually.

During my various formations, I came across the topic of "sports for old people". In more recent forms, this is referred to as 55+ or 60+ sports. I remember how one participant said she felt quite stigmatized by such labels, and many older people feel similarly ostracized. I for sure relate to their feelings. That is why I do not teach such formats at all. My courses and classes are open to anybody – and every participant will carry out the exercises as well as they can within the scope of their energy, vitality, and flexibility. Some use a chair for support in some exercises, and that is totally ok. In very much the same way, who finds the floor is too cold, puts an extra mat and/or a warm blanket under their back.

Trust me, from over 20 years of teaching Qigong and Yoga, I do know about all the smaller and bigger issues of the human body, as well as its aging process. Also, I have met a lot of younger people who suffer from various illnesses or have had accidents. I do wish to contribute to the common health and to us being and remaining an integrated society. It is in my interest and my philosophy to bring people together who love movement and health. I also appreciate the metaphysical or spiritual aspects of certain exercises. Through it, we can bring together the Yin and the Yang, and celebrate life and a joyful exchange together. The Five Tibetans are also called "Five Tibetan Rites", which points to the fact that their intention reaches well beyond just sports. "Rite" means more than "ex-ercise".

Overall, I have conceptualized each exercise in such a way that everybody can easily get into it. Every reader may decide for themselves, which of the exercises or parts thereof he or she wants to try out. Please always remain patient with your-self and treat your body and mind with care and mindfulness. Try feel your own body and self and be willing to follow their messages. For instance, someone with a stiff neck does not move their neck far back during the Third Tibetan. And no one wants to force the neck, or any other body part for that matter, through a barrier of pain. Do not endure! In case of difficulties, it is wise to only carry the exercise out to a rudimentary extent. And please, while I am at it, do the exercises in the correct order. Anyone who cannot perform one or more of the exercises, can simply leave them out, while maintaining the correct order of one through five.

On the Simplifications of the Tibetans in this Book

I will show smaller and easier steps for each Tibetan. This helps latecomers, the elderly, the ill, and recovering people to get a grip on the exercises. None of us is getting younger by the day. When watching videos on modern multimedia platforms such as YouTube or DailyMotion, one can find some pretty good presentations of the Five Tibetans. The average age of the person presenting them is thirty. At thirty we all moved easier and lither. Our physical condition and coordination are a lot better then.

The Tibetans are a sequence with a very long tradition, according to which older people were meant to enable their bodies and spirits to achieve a healthy state. I myself am approaching 60 now, and I want to demonstrate through my personal example how one can stay fit, healthy, forceful and mentally flexible until old age. It is exactly that which the Tibetans do for me, and that is why I think it is important that everyone gets a chance to learn them. In order for you to have a successful entry point I have written this book and made the corresponding videos.

From the bottom of my heart I want to recommend that you read other books on the subject as well. There is the booklet by Peter Kelder, who made the sequence known and popular in the West at the end of the 80s: "Ancient Secret of the Fountain of Youth". In order to get to know a subject well, it is recommended that you study several books and other teaching aids such as photos, videos, and DVDs. Maybe, you can come to a class personally.

My contribution herein is to present a revised form of the Five Tibetans – 2.0 – for all ages and states of health or fitness. I have over 20 years of experience with group and individual training, oftentimes with people, who have physical confinements or impairments. Yet, in my classes of Tai-Chi, Qi-Gong, and Yoga, all are welcome and can join. We always exercise together, and I support each one of my participants where they need it. The concept holds true for the entire book. Not all of you may need all the simplifying steps, but it is good to know that there will always be something which suits your needs exactly.

Right at the beginning I want to mention one important aid which concerns all the exercises. He or she who cannot – or not yet fully - carry out an exercise, is advised to do the following: Do this exercise in your mind's eye, i.e., close your eyes and envision yourself doing the exercise, before you even start moving. Another way would be to imagine someone else and how they are carrying out the exercise in a perfect way. The reason why this is so efficient is that, in Qi-Gong they have established that energies in the human brain are almost the same when they imagine doing the exercise compared to when physically doing it. At any rate, you will get a much clearer picture of flow and execution of an exercise, once you have memorized it in a mental way. Now, let us begin, and let me wish you all a lot of joy and health from it!

Creating the Best Place and Conditions for Practicing

Today, I hear often that exercises can be or even should be performable at any place such as the office. The idea is simply getting up and moving. Though I generally advocate exercising anywhere anytime because it just fits in with our modern way of living. Yet, the Tibetans are a different story, they are not primarily sport-like.

The Tibetans are not actually suitable for a little shake in-between two Zoom meetings. They want to unfold their value not only for the body, but also for mind and spirit. And that somehow takes some inner quietude as well as a certain amount of time which one is willing and able to put in. From my experience, you should give yourself at least 15-20 minutes for exercising and breathing techniques in the Tibetan rites.

You need a small even surface for exercising. That can be a carpet, a yoga mat or mat made from fibrea or other traditional or modern material, or simply the floor. Speaking of which, it is essential to make it comfortable enough for oneself. Coldness radiating from the floor does not bode well, for example. Some of the exercises are best performed barefoot. You should at least have a blanket ready or some warm socks. Most participants happily make use of the blanket (and a cushion) during the rest phases or even to keep their bodies warm when practicing in wintertime.

You want to wear light clothing, in which you can move lithely and easily. It is probably best to take your belt off because it impairs the bending of the upper body and hinders flowing movement in several of the exercises, especially for the Second Tibetan. He or she, who prefers to exercise in shoes, should try out light sneakers or gym shoes.

Music

There is one question people pose regularly: "Should I or may I have music in the background?" Yes, you may. I nevertheless advise against it – just like I did in my book on Qi Gong – because music always carries some sort of rhythm to us, which is why we love to use it for dancing. Yet, even the most relaxing music exerts an influence over our moving and breathing. While practicing deep exercises such as the Tibetan rites, I do not like such influences. Hence, I believe that without music, the Tibetans have a more rejuvenating and invigorating effect on the mind and body.

It is ultimately because the deeper effect can only unfold when one is focussed on oneself alone. Listening to music ties us to the external world instead of allowing us to concentrate on the inner and thus activate our self-healing forces on all levels. Moreover, it is quite decisive to find one's own breathing rhythm and make it as stable as possible. After weighing these positive effects that I gain only without music, I am happy to forgo a musical backdrop. Please try for yourself and find what's best for each one of you!

Preparation

Before exercising the Tibetans, one should not eat, let alone something heavy. It would strain our body and our flexibility. He or she who prefers to exercise in the morning, is recommended to do it with an empty stomach. Any (light) meal should happen at least 30 minutes before training. Moreover, it is best to not drink before the Tibetans, except half a glass of water or tea, both of which can be had in small sips also in between exercises, for instance after our repetitions of the 3rd Tibetan.

Under no circumstances should one practice the Tibetans under the influence of alcohol. We move and gather huge quantities of Qi (life energy) in our body and chakras via these exercises. Alcohol would totally destabilize this process. It goes without saying that this holds true for any other drugs, too. Especially given the mental and psychological implications of these exercises, one might want to clarify with one's general practitioner, if any medication may be contraindicated.

For myself I prepare a cup of green or Oolong tea, which I sip from in the rest -phases between the Tibetans. Then I turn my smartphone off and block other potential sources of noise or disturbances. While exercising I only belong to myself. This times serves my wellbeing, and I hold that very dear and precious. Hence, I make myself unavailable for any requests or talks.

Then, I shall begin to center myself.

Please first stabilize yourself and find peace and harmony before carrying out the rites. Relax. Make sure that you relax your jaw.

Breathe evenly, in and out.

Inhale. Then exhale again.

Breathe steadily and quietly. Notice how the phase of exhaling is slightly longer in order to increase the calming effect of your breathing on your entire body. Breathe with your nose only if possible.

Inhale. Exhale.

In. Out.

Now take your base stance, feet shoulder width apart, and you are now ready to begin with the First Tibetan.

Health Benefits of the Tibetan Exercises

The Five Tibetans do at the core help our spine. All five exercises gently stimulate the vertebrae, strengthen them, and increase their vibration. You may want to do the Tibetans before any other sports activity. The gentleness in which we perform all of them guarantees that the sensitive system of our spine is never strained. For this very reason, everyone is to carry out these exercises slowly. Please, never go past the limits of your own physical abilities. Never stress or overstrain your ligaments, sinews, vertebrae, or muscles here.

Our anatomical vertebrae have a spiritual counterpart in the Far East teachings. They call these spiritual energy wheels (or "vortices") or "Chakras". Chakra means a turning wheel of energy, a centre of energy which holds the entire human system of body and mind together. Moreover, they connect the inner world of the human with the outer world. With our exercises we gently stimulate these energetic centres, which rejuvenates them. They say that the ability of the chakras AND the anatomical vertebrae to vibrate and turn defines the true age of a human being.

The next important beneficiary of these exercises happens to be the endocrine system. The endocrine system comprises our human hormonal system and an entire network of glands throughout our body. These glands produce hormones and inject these into the blood stream, which transports them to all places in the body, even the most remote ones. Our hormonal system comprises many different signal substances, cells, and neighbouring glands. It is a whole system within our organ system, both of which are interlinked. Hormones directly and indirectly regulate our organ functions as well as our metabolic processes. They are a kind of messenger, which effect all neighbouring cells in a paracrine way, or they reach cells after having been released in an endocrine way into the blood stream.

Modern medicine, particularly research into aging, knows that the condition our hormone system is in, provides a direct mirror image of our true age. Some hormones such as testosterone decrease with aging. However, regularly exercising the Five Tibetans helps to slow down this process quite a bit. It may even be possible, like some of the ancient masters said, to reverse the aging process.

By doing the five exercises one at first normalizes, and then harmonizes the (turning/vibrating) velocity of the vertebrae as well as of our energy wheels, the chakras. In older and ill people, this mostly means increasing the speed at which they vibrate. This speed has been slowing down since we age. Along with the decrease in speed, what happens is a decrease in flexibility and vitality of the vertebrae, especially when we are ill. Sometimes, when we go through severe illness or trauma, the decrease in vitality may happen quite abruptly and seriously. In such cases, we age at an even more rapid and drastic rate, and all our organs and body parts become negatively affected.

One can neatly compare the re-vitalization process of the Five Tibetans with the formation of a vortex. This is because our anatomical vertebra swing and turn, too. Quite similar to the chakras they do not turn around, but they swing and they have a vibration. He or she who practices Qi -Gong for a while is aware of this moment in which we begin to feel our entire body vibrating. That shows that our body is filled with vital life -Qi (also referred to as breath, Prana, or universal energy). It is the same energy which supports us in mitigating all of our health-related issues such as with our intervertebral discs.

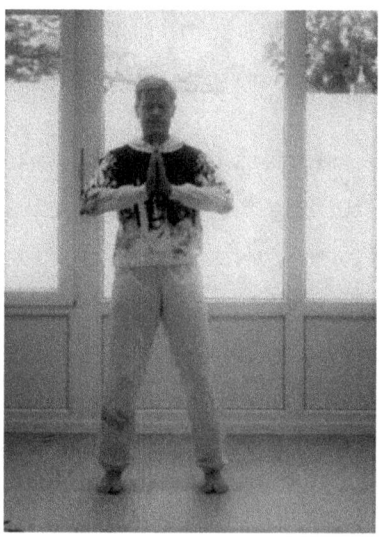

Please follow the breathing rhythm depicted herein to propel your individual health progress. This is because with proper breathing our bodies take in considerably higher amounts of oxygen, which simply equates to better overall health. More-over, our breathing becomes deeper, which helps our mind to relax and find its equilibrium. Only with that will come relax-ation, and without relaxation there is no healing. We may point to the fact that psychological illness is mostly related to states of unrest such as fear, phobias, or Angst. Interestingly, the base stance that I showed you (and which many of you know from my first Qi -Gong book), helps you to become in-wardly quiet, peaceful, and at ease. There are several varia-tions of the base stance, but their goal is always the same. Thus, please now take up the base stance and harmonize your breath.

Practical Tips for Your Exercises

For starters, I would like to recommend some things which are applicable to all 5 Tibetans. Create for yourselves a serene and harmonious space. Quietude should be all around. There should be no urgent business, no telephone calls, and no Facebook messages or notifications. Begin by simply standing within the quiet room, next to your mat.

He or she who prefers to swipe down the body – just like in Qi -Gong – in order to free themselves from old, stagnant energies, may do so by wiping their arms and legs in an outgoing direction two to three times. Use your left hand for the right arm and vice versa. Wipe your legs and upper body going towards the direction of your feet. One can easily carry out this small procedure within half a minute.

Afterwards, step on your mat, carpet or into a mentally determined place which represents your connection with the earth while practicing. Next to it put a cup of tea or a glass of water so that you don't need to go get it from the kitchen during the rest-phases. Personally, I put my tea on a little tea warmer with a burning tea light, which contributes to an overall quiescent atmosphere.

Do not strain your body in any of the five exercises. This includes maintaining regular breathing, i.e. no gasping, and no attacks of sweating or the like. The entire sequence requires you to exercise gently and evenly. Do not impose on yourself any duty of having to do any number of repetitions. It is our long-term goal to (re-) enable the body to repeat each Tibetan rite up to 22 times. Not more! But it is absolutely not required that you get there within 6 or 12 months. Please take into account your current physical and mental conditions, your personal state of fitness and health, as well as your feeling that day. Feel and sense your body and listen carefully to it. If for instance, your body tells you "it is enough now" after "only" four repetitions, then please follow your inner voice or intuition, even if yesterday you were able to do eight repetitions.

What is important is a certain continuity of practice, i.e., 12 minutes daily rather than 1 hour twice a week. Our vertebrae as well as our chakras want to continuously be accelerated, not over winded occasionally. It is worth mentioning that health is actually a process; we know how each of our processes suffers some setbacks every now and then.

If the outside temperature is hot, practice more slowly and with less muscle force than when the weather is colder. Indoor spaces should be neither too cold nor over-heated. On cold days, I prefer to wear a warm sweater at the beginning, which I then often take off after the second rite. Since breathing is so important, I have written the following extra paragraph on correct breathing during the exercises.

Breathing Correctly

Above all, it is important to breathe evenly and regularly. In. Out. In. Out. Just like in Qi Gong, breathing guides our movement. The same holds true for the Tibetans. Breathing guides moving, not vice versa. Never stop your breathing flow, not even when changing direction. For instance in the third Tibetan rite, when you start bringing the back up again, do not change your breathing. Always breathe evenly through your nose. This way your movements will become steady, quiet, and vigorous.

Breathing should happen as diaphragmatic breathing. Funnily enough, many people think that this means that the diaphragm also takes in oxygen, in addition to the lungs. In reality, the diaphragm is situated underneath the lungs and cannot itself "breathe". It actually consists of a group of muscles, which separate the chest cavity from the abdominal cavity. It is a sort of dome-shaped breathing muscle, which we can contract and expand, the latter of which helps the lungs to breathe in more deeply.

When we consciously expand the stomach area while breathing in, the diaphragmatic muscle expands to the outside and makes space for the lungs to expand, which fills them with more oxygen. Hence, the term "diaphragmatic breathing" means a muscular activity which enhances and deepens our breathing. He or she who does this outside of exercising will benefit their health immensely. Most people find it rather difficult, especially a lot of women. While performing the five

Tibetans, I strongly urge you to breathe like that. It supports the positive effects from the exercises quite a bit.

It is generally recommended to breathe through the nose on both the inhale and the exhale. Most people exhale with the mouth when practicing, but medical research has identified an increase in stress hormones as soon as one starts breathing through the mouth. This has to do with a very old part of our brain, the so-called amygdala, which is involved in what we call fight-or-flight situations and all lead to stress. In order to literally take all stress from our breathing, it is best to breathe with the nose during our exercises and rites. Try it out for yourselves. You should avoid any form of hectic breathing (e.g. impact respiration), which is always indicative of using too much force. People in the West, however, like that because they usually put themselves under pressure. Please refrain from that when practicing the Tibetans. None of the positive health effects can be forced, but they will unfold gradually, when one applies no more than max. 50% of one's power. Less is more!

The First Tibetan: Turning to the Right

The First Tibetan rite looks pretty easy. Turn around your own axis in a clockwise direction. The fact that this first exercise of the sequence is so very easy is actually the problem for most of the people that I teach it to. The Western mind fancies the thought that something has to be difficult or strenuous or else unpleasant for it to be beneficial. I see this kind of thing every Monday in class, when elderly gentlemen bend forward and want to touch the ground with their fingers, which is too much for most at that age. Most people make life unnecessarily difficult for themselves. Be good to yourself instead!

It is a fact that most of those who find the First Tibetan exercise too easy, will give up immediately at the second one, which is admittedly more difficult by structure and execution. Let me tell all of you: we are going to learn it together, and step by step. You will most likely get it right after a while. Therefore, train the grounding, the stability, and the breathing in the first Tibetan, then your force will surely unfold with the second rite.

Step into your special place now, feet pointing forward and approx. shoulder width apart. Lift your arms to the sides and stretch them out and away from the centre of your body. Palms are facing down to the earth. Keep your arms loose though; flex your muscles as little as possible. Your elbows should be slightly rounded so that Qi (energy) can flow unobstructed. Keep your shoulders loose. Actually, during my research for this book, I found quite a few pictures and videos, where people stretch their arms too straight and flex their shoulder muscles too much. Such a posture will only help speed up the spinning around, which is not what you are looking for. The correct position is therefore shown in the photo below on the left.

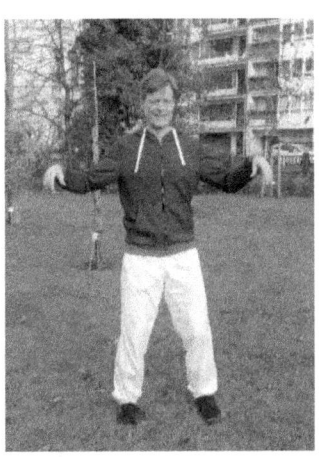 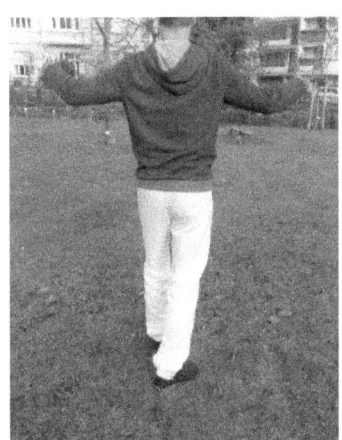

Then start spinning by putting your right foot slightly back and to the side (cf. photo above on the right). The position of the foot is at an angle of max. 45°. Your toes are pointing outward to the right side. It is important not to put the foot at a right angle to the left foot, which would only speed up the spinning movement. The opening to the right may actually be quite a bit less, such as 30° only. Please try it out and find how it is best for you in order to start spinning to the right.

By the way, many people have asked whether they should not "for equilibrium purposes" spin and turn the body around to the left also. Please, do not! The vibration of the vertebrae as much as of the chakras, when they are healthy, it to the right and not to the left. Therefore, it is best that you never turn to the left in this exercise. Amongst people who study the arts of energies or of spiritual healing, they find that turning around to the left will close the corresponding energy - channel. Since what we want to achieve is activating and boosting our energy system, I think that the only sensible thing to do is to open joints and chakras by spinning to the right.

The entire impulse for this exercise actually derives from the very first step we take. From there on in we simply put our feet alternatingly to the side and around. Always turn around your own axis in such a way that you get back into the exact position from which you started. Had you left a footprint in the starting basic stance, you would stand in those over again, after each circle around your own axis.

Spin slowly. Do not think of anything, if that's at all possible. Concentrate exclusively on the exercise and how it's done, in particular on your breathing. The correct way of performing the first Tibetan exercise is slowly, really very slowly. Yet, one can still get dizzy or even nauseous. If that happens, most teachers will tell you to fix your eyes on one specific spot in your space and keep it there, such as an object of art or a vase. That's the way dancers or figure skaters do it, but this argument is wrong and counterproductive. Whoever spins around may get dizzy, at least at the beginning. That is quite normal. It reveals that your vertebrae, joints, and chakras still vibrate at a pretty low frequency. We must totally respect that; hence, we should refrain from overcoming this by force or "musts" or tricks. On the contrary, I strongly suggest lowering your speed, when you become dizzy. Or else, stop with this exercise, at least for today.

In the beginning, it is absolutely ok to only spin three times. Then, very carefully and slowly increase the number of repetitions respecting your age and state of health. Always listen carefully to your body. Be mindful. Follow the principle of mindfulness (cf. Tippach "Opening the 9 Gates"). Trust me, you will reach your goal more speedily by spinning more slowly, and you will stop dizziness or nausea completely.

Another thing you should avoid completely is the phenomenon of the "ecstasy of the whirling dervish". In shamanic cultures, they all know how the medicine man of their village spins around for as long as it takes to fall into some kind of trance or ecstasy, which is supposed to lie outside of our normal reality. I thinks it is self-evident why when practicing the Five Tibetans, we do not at all aim at such trance states, but actually strictly avoid them.

Common Errors and Corrections for the First Tibetan

Some of the most commonly made errors when practicing the First Tibetan, are the following:

- The spinning is too fast

- The spinning happens abruptly or even in fits and starts

- The spinning movement is uneven

- One changes positions and moves around

- One wants too much and spins too often

- People drop their hands or lift them above shoulder height

- The shoulders convulse

It is correct to spin evenly and slowly with small side and backward steps. It is absolutely ok to stop every now and then for a shorter break, in particular when you have just started your practice. For that purpose, it is ok to restart two or three times. It is, for instance, quite an in-between achievement to reach six spinning movements while subdividing them into 2 times 3.

Especially for older people, or ill or recovering exercisers, it is recommended to add some moments of rest between repetitions, on top of the resting -phases between the individual rites. Like I mentioned earlier, it is best to increase the number and intensity of the individual exercises only gradually and quite slowly. Every time you move on, I advise you to check in with your current physical condition and make the required adjustments.

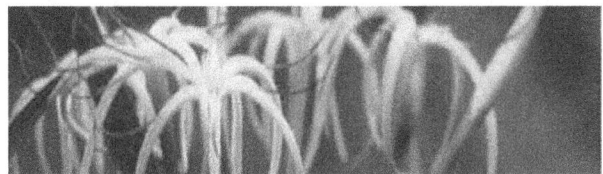

He or she who spins too fast, easily loses their balance. One literally uproots oneself by the power of one's spin. Then, one loses one's composure and staggers through the room. That shows that one is still exercising with too much force or wanting to achieve too much too quickly. Slow down! One who starts skidding still has too little "grounding". Call it steadfastness, stability, or earth connectedness – whichever expression you may prefer. But one thing is for sure, namely, that our feet connect us with mother Earth. This connection needs to be strong indeed, so that your body can strengthen, and you become healthy or stay that way. That is why I recommend standing still in the base stance before even starting the spinning movement. Become aware, or remind yourself again, of the importance of your connection with the ground. Become firm in your consciousness and thus in your stance.

The outward stretching of your arms adds to your stability. Keep that up throughout the exercise. Should you feel your arms become tired, it is about time to rest or probably even stop the repetitions of the first Tibetan rite for today.

The same is true in case your shoulders begin convulsing, cramping, or you feel compelled to pull them upward. The posture of the arms serves to stabilize your body, your equilibrium, and the straightening of your spine. Altogether, this exercise is more difficult than at first glance. If necessary, one should strengthen one's musculature by a Qi –Gong -exercise called "push the mountain to the side" (cf. Tippach "Opening the 9 Gates"). Ultimately, our goal is to be able to do twenty-two repetitions.

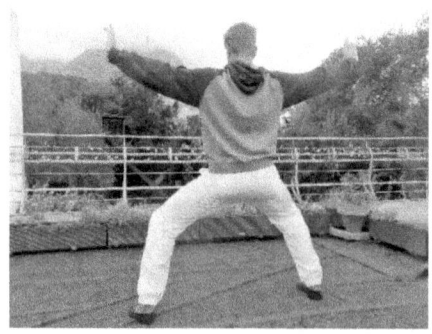

Transition from the First to the Second Tibetan

We can consider the smooth changing over from one Tibetan exercise to the next to be an art in itself, even though most teachers hardly ever address it. Towards the end of this book I dedicate an entire chapter to this topic. At this point, I would like to give special attention to something which older or ill people should apply to the in-between –exercises -phases. The reason for this is because we gain a healthy increase of vibration during the individual exercises, which we naturally want to conserve for its long-term benefits. However, through incorrect changing-over to the next exercise, one stands to lose quite a bit of one's achievements. Imagine, as an extreme example making a telephone call or surfing the internet instead of properly resting.

Let us assume, you have already managed 8 spins and have reached your starting position again. Stay there standing with your arms stretched for a couple of moments. Then, if it feels right to you, lower your hands to a middle height and relax, without any flexing of your musculature, your body remaining entirely loose. If you need to sit down, do so. It is also an excellent idea to use the Qi -Gong basic stance during this phase. Your hands are loose here too. (cf. photo below on the right).

Most teachers that I have met teach a slightly different version of this relaxing stance. According to them, one holds one's palms together in front of the chest, as if you were praying (cf. photo below on the left). This may feel relaxing to some, and it is actually not wrong. Personally, I have no positive view on this alternative, though. Try it out for yourself; see what feels better to you. Most people in my classes say that this stand leads to tensions in their neck and/or upper arms. That is exactly what you will avoid, when your hands are lowered, loose and relaxed.

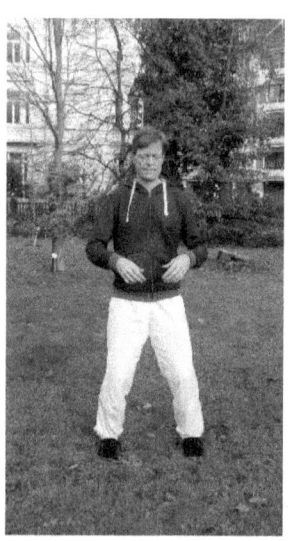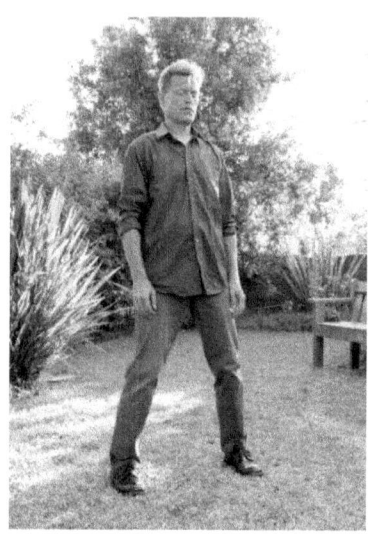

I would like to draw your attention to another important fact. In the quiet stance after performing the first Tibetan, something else will happen that is actually quite decisive! Feel your body and begin to perceive it for yourself. One participant in my workshops once expressed it spot-on: "It feels as if, despite me being in a resting position, the vertebrae (chakras) in my back are still spinning around". That is exactly so. The positive health effects have started to kick in!

One need not be clairvoyant for this perception at all, or even make something up. The more you exercise, the more such perceptions will become quite "normal" for you, which simply means that you are beginning to perceive your body on its energetic levels. Even though this is not necessary, it is quite a pleasant side effect which shows you that you are making good progress.

This further rotation in the back or in the entire body can go on for several minutes in advanced practitioners. At the beginning when the experience is quite new, I would recommend really enjoying this and feeling how your body undergoes vitalization and self-healing. Later, one should pay less attention to it; one should be conscious of it, but no longer focus on it.

You can rest in between the rites, if that is necessary, by sitting or lying down. However, please carefully weigh up before making a decision. Needing a lot of rest between the rites may suggest that you probably overdo it with the exercises themselves. That would not further your health at all. It is better to apply less force, max. 50% with no need for extensive breaks or rest-phases between the Tibetan exercises.

Indulge in a sip of tea, if you like.

Or some water.

However, refrain from eating.

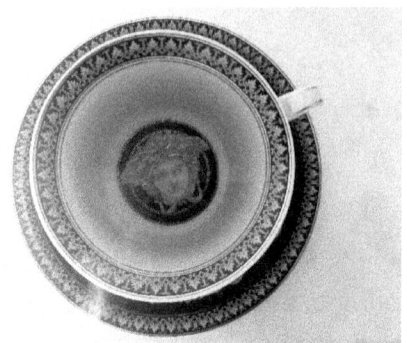

Should you feel dizzy or even nauseous during or after the first Tibetan rite, despite all preventative measures, please do wait for this emotion to pass completely. Only then is it safe to start with the second Tibetan exercise.

The "Sixth" Tibetan?

We also want to address some spiritual secrets around the Tibetans. There is indeed a so-called sixth Tibetan rite. In truth, it actually is an "exercise" which goes together with each of the Five. For the advanced student, it is possible to include an added mantra. "Advanced" means that you can perform each of the rites harmoniously and without further having to think about how to do them. He or she who wants to use the additional exercise presented by Kelder as the sixth, would then consider the mantra as the seventh Tibetan.

Kelder's version of the sixth exercise is meant to spark the so-called "Kundalini" energy. I hear this kind of teaching a lot. The mere formulation shows, with all due respect, that there is a lot of ignorance around this topic. *Kundalini* is not so much a form of energy, but rather an additional chakra, which is opened in very few people. Trying to handle it is actually quite dangerous. Trying to access this immense power is definitely the wrong way for beginners and even most advanced students.

The correct "Sixth" Tibetan is an accompanying mantra for one or all of the other rites. *Mantra* means an affirmation or positive sentence, which we monotonously repeat (inwardly) while performing the rites. Such a mantra can help deepen your experience and also autosuggest positive things to your consciousness. However, let me be clear on this: It is not a sign that one is advanced in the Tibetans, nor in spiritual things in general. It is absolutely not necessary to repeat any mantras with the exercises in order to make progress. It is also definitely not necessary to say them aloud. It is sufficient to formulate them internally or think them or hum them. Personally, I do this only from time to time just like I practice the so-called "healing sounds" in Qi Gong very sparsely. It is mostly a matter of how one feels on a given day. One possible beautiful mantra for the First Tibetan is:

"My movements are free, without intentions, and considerate"

He or she who prefers it a bit more "spiritual" may prefer:

"I am open for the cosmic/ Godly/all-encompassing energy (Qi)". Or, "I am open for the (Godly) love".

Quite a few participants told me that they would like to accompany one or the other exercise with the famous sound "OM". That, I feel, is a pretty good idea.

Everyone needs to feel and decide for themselves if any mantra adds something good for them, or whether it actually touches their heart. If not, simply drop it! Please do not feel obliged to speak it or think it while practicing your Tibetans.

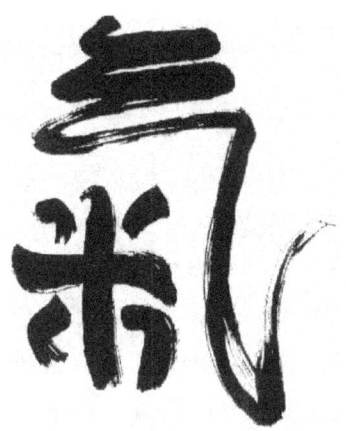

The Second Tibetan: Lifting your Legs and Neck

Many people want to give up right away when they see the second exercise. A lot of older people even believe that "this is not for them anymore". I will have to admit that the Second Tibetan is not a simple exercise, but it is doable. I have structured this in such a way for you – and in particular for you older or weaker people – that you can learn it step by step. I have incorporated in these steps all of my insights gained in workshops and seminars. I always give every participant the opportunity to present his or her specific problems with an exercise. In addition, each one of them helped me, quite gradually, to get a grip on my endeavour to make this second Tibetan exercise accessible for all.

The main health effect of the Second Tibetan is due to a short, gentle stretch of the spine. In doing so, we extend the vertebrae like cymbals on a thread, which you can find around Buddhist monasteries. The cymbals start singing through the gentle stretch of the thread. The singing sound equals the health-promoting vibration I have mentioned before, and which happens to the anatomical vertebrae as well as to the chakras. You will improve your health a lot by doing the second Tibetan, so please try. Should you have trouble, just refer to the individual steps that I am going to outline in a moment. Be patient and muster some courage, you'll succeed for sure!

The basic physical movement of the second Tibetan consists of bringing up your head and legs from a lying position, breathing in, and then breathing out and bringing them gently back down to the ground. Please also refer to the **videos** on my **PATREON** page. Keep your hands relaxed next to your hips, palms facing up (for beginners). This exercise requires comfortable clothing; personally, I have to take off my belt for this one. For all of the following in-between -steps it is totally ok to put your hands (or only your thumbs if you prefer) under your buttocks (instead of next to the hips) in order to stabilize your posture. This facilitates lifting your legs quite considerably. When progressing, you will want to put your hands next to your body and lift your legs through the force stored in your body centre (in Qi -Gong we call it *Dan Tien*).

Making Progress in Five Small Steps

You will find a description of the complete exercise in step down down below. Let us now begin simplifying it by looking at partial steps. Please advance exactly according to your own needs. After the in-between rest -phase after the First Tibetan, lie down on your back with your legs stretched out and your arms resting next to your body. If you haven't used a mat this far, now is a good moment to unroll it because under no circumstances should your back get cold.

Step One

Lie quietly on your back and relax. Now lift your head a bit and bend your toes towards your shins (cf. first photo below). I guess you can feel right away the gentle stretching like the soft pulling of a thread on your spine. This can already relax the spinal canal in quite a pleasant way, and it also kicks off the vibration of the vertebrae. In addition, even if you cannot yet lift your leg(s), for instance because you injured your leg muscles, this first step is very beneficial for your health.

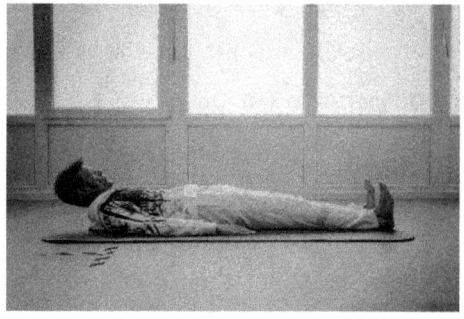

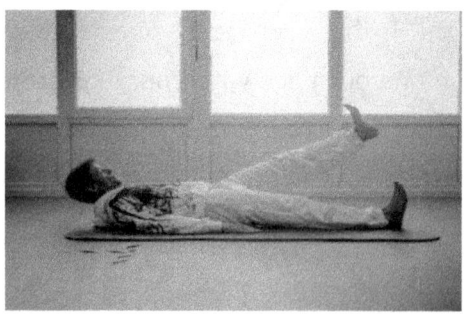

Step Two

Leave you head slightly elevated. Please do not lift your head very far, let alone with a full stretch of the neck so that you would be able to look straight ahead. Lift your legs alternatingly, starting with the left leg, then the right one (cf. photo above on the right). Do this as slowly as possible. Breathe in while you lift the leg and breathe out while putting it gently back on the ground. Between each lifting movement, lie still on the floor with legs and neck fully relaxed for at least one full breath in and out.

Step Three = Further Facilitation of Step Two

It is decidedly not easy to lift a leg straight up while lying down. This is due to resulting high tension in the hip-, stomach-, and thigh areas. Many students to whom I taught the Five Tibetans were not able to do this in the beginning. Therefore, I would like to suggest beginning with the following easier alternative:

Starting from your lying position, draw one knee towards your body bending it slightly upwards. Should this be too difficult for your current health condition, please just put one foot next to the knee of the other leg, which remains on the ground. Start with your left leg. Put your left foot next to the right knee (cf. first photo below). If you wish, you may breathe in and out one more time in this position. Then, bring your left leg up further starting with your left foot. Do not attempt to bend the leg in a right angle (90°) with your sole

47

pointing to the sky. You may improve this in smaller steps later on (cf. second photo below).

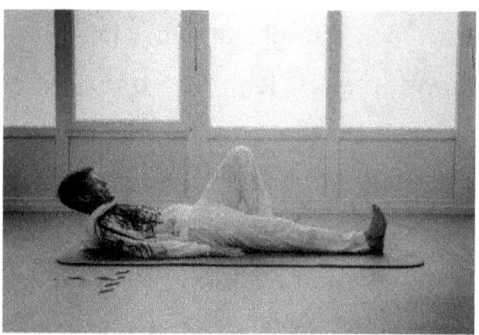

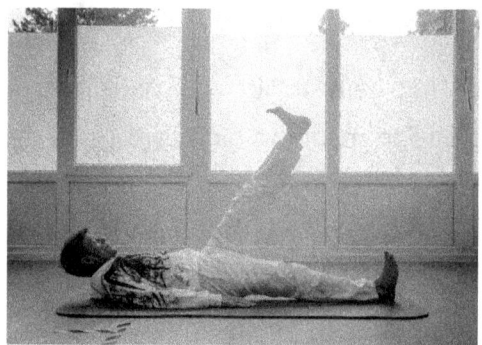

The important thing here is to maintain the correct breathing rhythm, i.e., inhaling when lifting the leg and exhaling when bringing the leg gently back down. When adding in the next step, please make sure that your breathing stays correct. What could easily happen is that you breathe in with the first bending of the leg, and then are tempted to breathe out when lifting the leg further up. That would be wrong, though.

You may experience problems with your back; especially the lower back can get tense or even painful. This corresponds probably with a lack of muscle power in your back. The Second Tibetan does indeed help to build up muscles in the lower back area, but it can take a while, which is why one must never overdo it, especially not when beginning the training. Moreover, you should under no circumstances inflict pain upon yourself!

He or she who prefers the position with their knees bent should consider doing the same bending on the way back to the ground. This brings about another facilitation and relief. Practically speaking, you can add the bending of your knee when lifting one leg at a time (step two) as well as when you already lift both legs together (step four). Bending our knees on the way down is anatomically a lot less strenuous for the leg musculature. This way you prevent the danger of over-straining your leg muscles and of back pains.

Step Four

This step is very important for those experiencing problems with the second rite. Herein, we lift both legs simultaneously. First, do it as described in step three, namely bend the knees (cf. first photo below), then begin lifting your legs further up. Please always remember to inhale when lifting the legs *and* the head at the same time. From the bent position of the knees, lift the legs further up by first stretching them. It is more than ok if your final position is not the right angle of 90° (cf. second photo below).

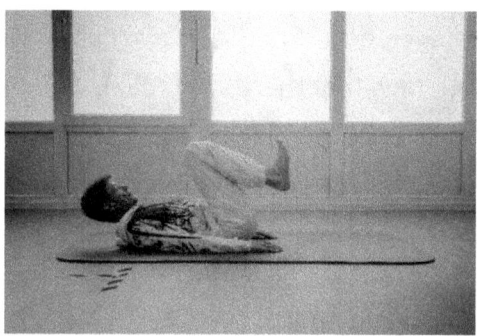

You can measure your progress by several factors. Firstly, you begin to succeed more and more in lifting your legs. Secondly, you will feel better and you will want to do more repetitions. Keep breathing correctly, inhale on the way up, and exhale on the way down. Accessing the power in your body centre will give you a notion of how much energy there really is within you. It may surprise you in a very positive way.

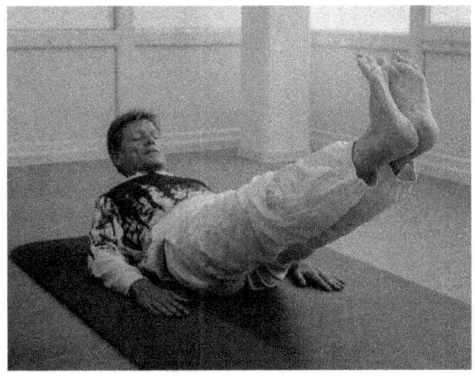

Step Five: The Complete Second Tibetan

Now you are prepared to perform this Tibetan fully and in the traditional way. You can be proud of yourself because this is quite an achievement. Be assured that your health benefits greatly from it. He or she, who can do this exercise in one go (without interruption or additional breathing) can easily deduct 10-15 years from their "passport age". Your real biological age is already reduced! The ultimate secret of the Tibetans is that they not only slow down the aging process, but also in the end start to even reverse it.

Lie down on the ground. Breathe in lightly, lifting your head and bending your toes towards your shin. From your body centre, gather force enough to lift both legs up to a 90° angle breathing in. Then, start breathing out and brings your legs slowly and gently back to the ground. Remain in this relaxed position for one (or more, if you need) full breathing cycle. Then repeat the exercise over, and up to 22 times. The more advanced practitioner, who has already strengthened their heart and lungs, won't even need the additional breathing cycle when lying down. It may take approx. 1-2 years for you to be able to perform this Tibetan in such a way. He or she who has mastered this, has already mostly stopped their aging process.

Several participants expressed how they felt that the final position, i.e., legs up in a 90° angle and the neck lifted, reminded them of an "open blossom". Personally, I am not much of a poet, but I do like this image a lot. Should it appeal to you too, then maybe you want to inwardly accompany the exercise with the following inner mantra: "I am open like a (lotus) flower for Love/the Godly".

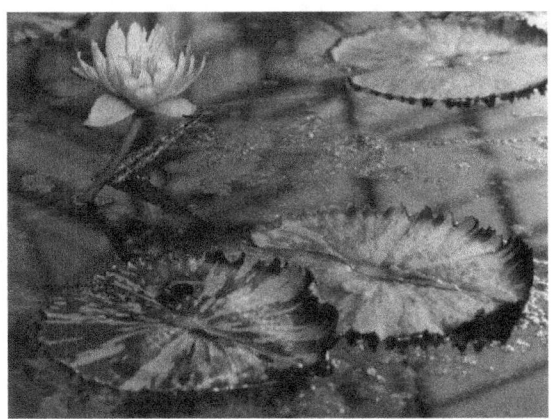

Advanced Alternative

My Qi -Master in Taiwan taught me this alternative. Traditional teaching is quite aware that before Yoga and Qi- Gong parted ways, there was an even older system of exercises for body and mind. The Five Tibetans may very well be part of this older system from the Himalayas. He told me to put the back of my hands on the floor so that my palms faced towards the Sky. When lowering the legs, one then also turns the hands around so that the palms face towards the Earth. I believe that we should never aim at any specific results. Moreover, I don't want anybody to put themselves under pressure or expectations. Therefore, I specifically abstain from describing the additional effects of the hand posture for mind and body. Those of you who have come this far are certainly able to sense and perceive which parts of an exercise can help create which form of energies. I can entrust you fully with your physical and mental sensations and perceptions.

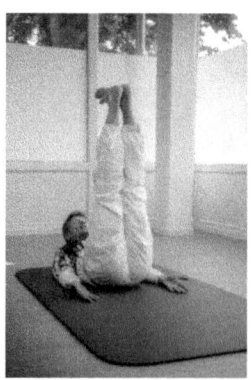

Common Errors and Corrections for the Second Tibetan

Commonly made mistakes when performing the Second Tibetan exercise are listed below. At this juncture, I would also like to extend an invitation to all readers. He or she who finds further mistakes, or is unsure of the correct performance, simply contact mail@dr-tippach.de – so I can clarify and maybe even bring it into this book in a next edition.

- Buttocks and/or hips are lifted up together with the legs. It is correct, though, to push both against the ground, especially when lifting the legs.

- People often forget to tense and bend their toes before lifting the legs.

- While tensing one's toes, often one forgets to inhale. However, the bending of the toes and feet is the beginning of the next upward movement. Hence, please begin to breathe in at the same time. The actual impulse for lifting the legs comes from your heels. One starts lifting one's legs from the heels by tensing and bending one's toes towards the shines.

- The neck gets tensed too much and/or moved up too high. Younger or over-ambitious people, who want to achieve a lot by demanding as much as possible from their bodies, often make this mistake. This is, however, the wrong starting point and attitude. We must never force our vertebrae, neither medically nor spiritually. Instead, we may only gently stimulate them. The vortices around our energetic centres, the chakras, do function as interfaces for our other levels, bodies (such as our emotional or spiritual bodies) and the etheric (cf. the term "Ätherleib" according to Rudolf Steiner) dimensions.

- Even though we aim at bringing our legs up to a 90° angle (some very flexible people can do it even a bit further than that), at the beginning 45° is perfectly fine. Practice the second rite regularly and thus your sinews will improve in strength so that you can stretch up your legs more and more. But please, never overstrain yourself!

- The upward movement of the legs is often too abrupt. Rather, one should inhale very gently and guide the legs upward in the same gentle way. Abrupt movement here happens mostly due to a lack of muscle force in the thighs and/or in the centre of the body. I suggest that for as long as your movement is abrupt, you simply lift your legs less or decrease the number of repetitions of this Tibetan.

- The downward movement of the legs is too abrupt. I suggest exhaling very gently while you move your legs back down, and from a lesser angle.

The Third Tibetan: Bending our Neck Backwards

Some call the Third Tibetan the "backward spine-stretcher". Just like in Qi- Gong, I am not fond of the flowery names of some of the exercises. Therefore, I would like to drop this "anatomical monster" of an expression. Let us simply call it the third rite. And now, let us begin exercising it together. The third exercise contributes to a wonderful gentle stretching of our spine, and thus strengthens our back and our thighs quite nicely.

The basic idea of the third rite is to bend your spine gently forth and back. The movement to the back is a lot deeper than to the front. This also stimulates all our vertebrae and makes them "elastic" and flexible. Our anatomical vertebrae consist of hard discs and soft interspaces between them. He or she suffering from slipped or herniated discs has most often used up the softer parts; the harder parts rubbing against one another is the main cause of pains in this area. The reason is usually that the person always moved in a "hard" way, took upon herself heavy burdens, and over-strained their Yang at the cost of the softer, female Yin-parts. It would therefore be a pretty bad idea to extend this kind of non-equilibrium to this exercise. Please never perform the third rite with great willpower! Rather, apply gentleness and mindfulness, namely with respect to your discs and vertebrae. Do not wish for "achievements" here!

The Third Tibetan focuses on our spine, whose anatomical importance includes protecting our nerve pathways, which are the most important connections of the body with the brain. The structure of the spine represents the overall human connection between the above and the below, Heaven and Earth. The exercise itself enhances our flexibility, openness, permeability, and the exchange of the poles or the above and the below. Hence, we activate our vertical energies and further our physical and spiritual existence at the same time. In Qi-Gong, we call the poles the male (above) and the female (below). This exercise gives us a chance to energetically unite Heaven and Earth in our human bodies.

After the resting -phase between the second and third rite, sit down on your calves. I advise you to use a mat here, or even an additional cushion in order to not hurt the knee joints. The best way of getting into this position is to kneel down with your toes touching the ground – much in the same way we did this as children using our calves and feet as the sitting surface. The bridge of our feet points to the earth and we actually sit mostly on our feet. This is in itself not so easy because knees and feet are to set about shoulder width apart (cf. photo below). I urge you strongly to get used to this sitting position before you even begin with the actual exercise. Similar to Qi Gong, we need a safe and stable base position, without which our performance will lack precision and ultimately, we will miss out on many health benefits as well.

Should you need an additional layer to cushion your weight, try an extra mat or a soft blanket underneath your knees. It is so good to feel how we strengthened our sinews and ligaments in the exercises before. Otherwise, this mixture between sitting and squatting would be too difficult. He or she who still experiences difficulties should warm up for this exercise with some simple knee bends.

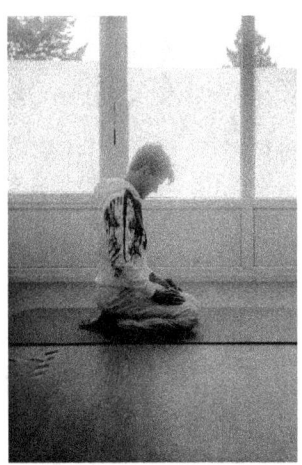

Next, put your hands on your lower back for support with the fingers pointing to the earth and the hands being slightly angular. Supporting your back serves to protect your upper body and in particular your vertebrae from strain and injury. Moreover, through the slight pressure of the balls of the hands you gently stimulate your kidneys and thus energize them. Keep your hands in this position from beginning through end of the third rite including all repetitions (photo below on the left).

N.B.: Over time, some points of discussion have developed around the Tibetan exercises. One of them is about the position of the hands. Some recommend putting the hands on the back of the thighs. This is also a supportive position, but in my eyes less effective than the above-mentioned one. It may be more suitable for people with disproportionately long arms. Every one of you can try out what feels best. I do not teach the latter alternative because it only supports the back indirectly. Moreover, one misses out on the energetic benefits for the kidneys (photo below on the right).

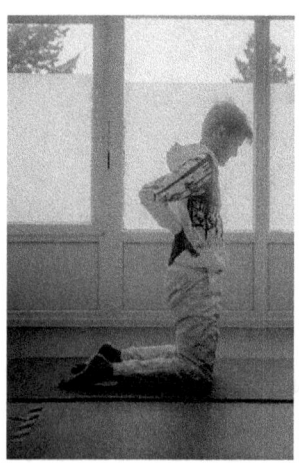 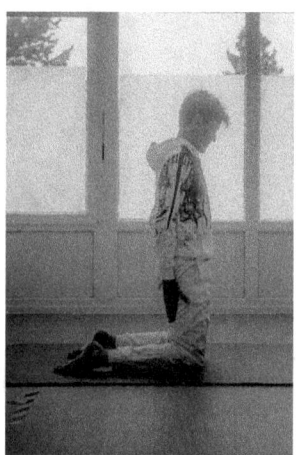

Begin the third rite by exhaling. Remain in your starting position, "sitting on your feet". Gently breathe in and out. Then, exhaling, you bend the neck slightly forward. Don't overdo it! More experienced practitioners may extend this first movement so that their chin touches the chest. However, there are no medals or rewards for this, and it is neither necessary nor vital. Remember that the Tibetans aim at gently stretching the spine, like a thread with cymbals. Through each light pull at the neck or in the coccyx area, the cymbals sound and your vertebra vibrate. No anatomical peak performance is ever helping with that.

Then, stretch your thighs so that your body forms an "L-shape". The bridges of the feet remain on the ground and so do the knees. The entire rest of the body draws itself up. Come back to this upright position each time your breathing-cycle restarts. This happens without lowering it back into the sitting position, which one gets into only once one has carried out all repetitions.

Start the core exercise movement lifting your neck back up while beginning to inhale. Remember, bending your neck for-ward went together with an exhaling -phase. Now guide your upper body gently backwards while breathing in. Your hips remain in a stable position. Many people try at first to push their hips forward, but that is incorrect. Bend your upper body gently back (photo above on the right) which stretches your "cymbals"/vertebrae gently and helps them vibrate in a healthy way. For beginners, I suggest limiting this exercise to 3-4 repetitions. Gather some facts concerning how far you can bend back without incurring pain or discomfort. Go easy! (cf. photo below on the left)

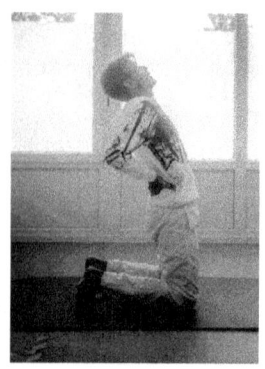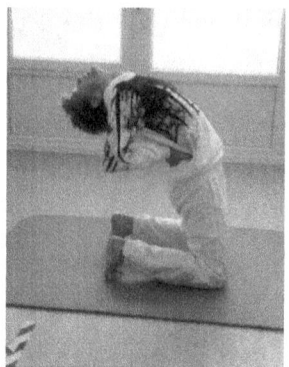

I emphasize this because many of my participants are almost in shock when watching me perform this bending my upper body and neck pretty far back. Doing so is safe only for very advanced practitioners or professionals (cf. photo above on the right).

He or she who is already in a good physical condition and knows for sure that they can bend and stretch their back safely, will begin to extend the movement quite naturally than would be good for a beginner. Advanced students may also bring their head further back.

Suitable mantras accompanying this exercise are:

"The Above and the Below in me
are in loving exchange"

"I am equally well connected with the
Above and the Below"

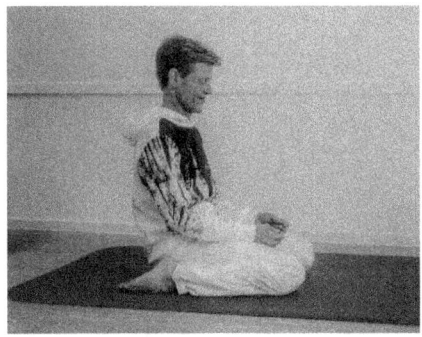

How to Breathe Correctly during the Third Tibetan

The inhaling -phase synchronizes with the bending back-wards. It is important not to breathe in bursts. Bending the back also compresses the lungs which makes it a bit difficult to inhale anyways. Hence, many practitioners tend to ab-ruptly breathe in at the beginning of the bending movement. However, it is best to gently and evenly fill your lungs, which requires quite a bit of attention and experience.

Alternative for Beginners

When starting to practice this exercise, you should bend the neck and back visibly less forward and backwards. For this Tibetan we need quite a stable and strong musculature, which we often lack when aging or in recovery. Without sufficient muscular force, our lower vertebra have to carry all of our weight. Our lumbar vertebrae carry the main burden. That is why I strongly suggest beginning with a very gentle and light bending of the back (cf. photo below).

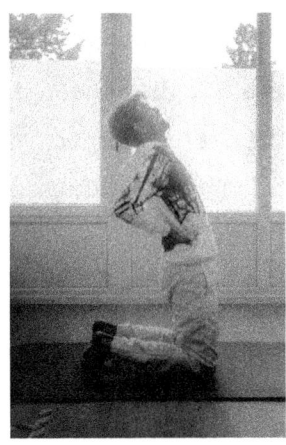

Common Errors and Corrections for the Third Tibetan

During the course of more than 20 years of teaching, I've seen and corrected in cooperation with my participants the following common mistakes people make when performing the second rite:

- The force for bending backwards comes from the lumbar vertebrae or the lower back in general. Unfortunately, this reverses the pulling effect on the spine. The third exercise wants you to stretch your vertebrae from the top of the spine and "pull" it gently. Therefore, it is correct to allow the movement to come from the neck up. At the start, the neck actually remains stiff and non-bent. Only practitioners who feel comfortable enough with this exercise should bend the neck slightly at the end of the bending movement of the back.

- People often get the toe positions wrong by putting the toes to the sides when sitting on their feet. The reason being mostly that the kneeling position is still too strenuous, e.g., it feels as if the ligaments in the thighs and/or the calves are over-stretched. The correct position is to point all five toes to the ground. You "sit" on your feet so to speak, with your soles pointing upwards.

- Another common error is to begin exhaling too late. Older people especially want to bring their back up again and then begin to breathe out, or they start on the way back up. It is correct to inhale the whole way downwards (i.e., while bending the back backwards) and exhale on the way up. There is an important principle of breathing, which is also valid in Qi -Gong: The breathing guides the movement, and not the other way around. We can say that the "movement flows through the breathing". Therefore, please try to change over from inhaling to exhaling as your upper body reaches the furthest extent backwards. Keep breathing out until your neck is bent forward, or even until you touch your chest with your chin. Then restart the breathing -cycle, bring your neck back up while inhaling and so forth.

The Transition between the Third and Fourth Tibetan

There exist several methods of transition between the third - and the fourth rites. Usually, it is taught to rest your upper body on the ground after your final repetition. You can also lay your weary upper body down on the backs of the hands that you have put on the floor in front of you.

This is a good and comforting position. However, for practically all beginners, this proves too difficult. Should you experience difficulties sitting on your calves and feet, you cannot expect to be able to perform what's actually a yoga -exercise called "the leaf" AND to relax at the same time (cf. the photo in the final section of this book). I have never seen that happening.

I therefore demonstrate in an extra chapter which other possible transitions there are between the Tibetans. For now, you can either sit down in a fashion quite similar to how you started this exercise, namely, on your feet and calves. If you are not yet able to sit in this way, you have probably figured out by now how which position suits you to begin this exercise. Simply rest your hands in your lap. Relax! Any position which does not involve bringing your upper body further down is good at this time. Make sure there is neither pain nor strain in your thighs and calves.

Alternatively, simply sit on the floor. Either stretch out your legs, bend them, or rest them on the floor, for instance in a

45°-angle to your left- and to your right-hand side. By bending your knees in this seated position, you reduce the strain on your sinews even further. He or she who does still not feel comfortable (and I have seen that a lot at this point) can just sit on a comfortable chair with a back rest. What is most decisive at this juncture is to give your back some time to adjust, relax, and re-organize itself.

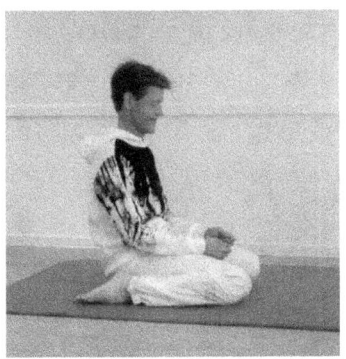 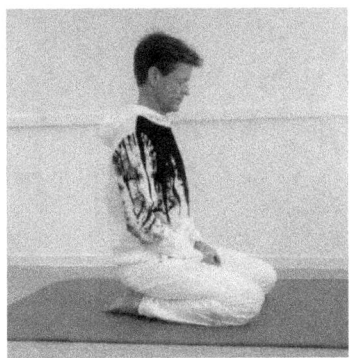

The more practice and fitness one has gained over time, the more one will tend to shorten the time in -between the exercises until you actually drop them (almost) completely. At this moment in time, however, you want to make sure to be in a position where you can harmonize your breathing cycle and relax your entire body. This is so important here because the fourth rite seems to be the most challenging one.

The Fourth Tibetan: Push up your Pelvis

In the long run, I believe that the fourth Tibetan rite is the most difficult one. That is because one has to combine several physical elements with one's breathing: upward movement while inhaling, downward movement with exhaling, and alternating between tension and relaxation of one's entire musculature during one exercise. I am speaking here in my function as trainer of the German Sports Association: this is quite demanding! I promise to guide all of you in six safe steps towards a correct method of performing the fourth Tibetan rite.

The core issue of this exercise is a stretching of the spine (remember, the thread with the resonating cymbals hanging from it) and getting one's chakras to vibrate healthily. I deem it beneficial, if not necessary, to do this exercise barefoot. In just socks, there is too much danger of sliding. Remember that a solid basic stand is essential for all exercises, particularly in this one.

First, bring your feet into the right position. The basic idea of this rite is an inversion of your body. From practicing Yoga, you may be familiar with several forms of inversion such as handstands or headstands, or the so-called "candle". The idea behind all of them is to invert all energy currents within the body at least once a day. This includes letting your lymph fluids run in the opposite direction for a while, as well as anything passing through your intestines. This helps unblock the passageways and also stimulates the "correct" flow of fluids and energies within you. Here, we begin in a sitting position, your hands and feet rest next to your body, both about shoulder -width apart.

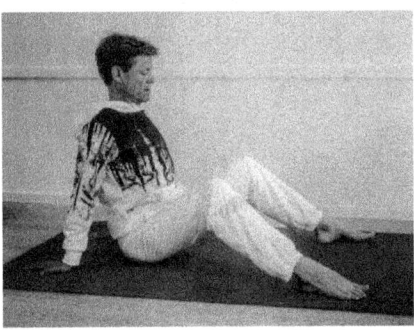

Sit as upright as possible, and on the floor or your mat. Put your feet shoulder -width apart. Yoga practitioners are probably familiar with the anatomical term for the position that we want to get into, the "table -position". It's called this because your back is supposed to be straight as a table. So, go from sitting to the table -position and then follow with a gentle lowering of the body back to the initial sitting position. Hands rest at the side of the body, palms facing down and fingers pointing to the front. Exhale in the sitting position. Then start to breathe in. Push your body forcefully upwards, lift your pelvis/buttocks and your upper body until you reach the table position (cf. photo below).

In the final position, your feet point forward, and your lower legs form a straight angle of 90°. From your knees up to the top of your head, your entire body now forms a straight line. This proves time and again to be very difficult for older people, beginners, and recovering people. Since one is looking up to the ceiling, the body and its posture easily destabilize. All of which makes me want to describe the whole thing to you in a simplified version, which I will do step-by-step below:

Step One: Bringing One's Buttocks Up

First, push your buttocks up, coming from the seated position. However, leave your upper body and your head on the ground. This way you will succeed in strengthening the muscles which are essential for performing the Fourth. This is in general beneficial to your power and health. Inhale while pushing the buttocks up, then exhale while bringing them safely and gently back to the ground. Remain stretched out and relaxed for several breaths. Harmonize your breathing and rest on the ground.

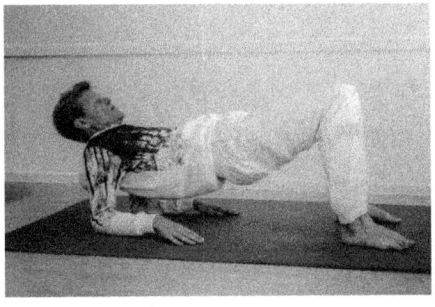

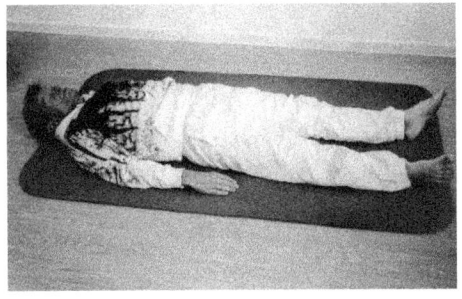

Step Two: Pushing up Your Upper Body

Once you have trained for a couple of days or even weeks to push your buttocks up with the force of your hands and feet. Now, what you do is push up both buttocks and your upper body. At this point, it is not important whether you reach the 90° angle or the "table position". I suggest you do not yet lower the neck. Rather, for now keep on watching straight ahead of you (cf. photo above). This position is a lot less challenging. Moreover, it helps you maintain stability and staying in control by keeping a general overview of where you are and what is happening around you. While pushing upwards, please inhale. Then lower your buttocks and your upper body again, exhaling. Remain seated for a bit and do a couple more relaxing and soothing breaths. This way, you get accustomed to the entire movement of the fourth rite step by step controlling your breathing rhythm.

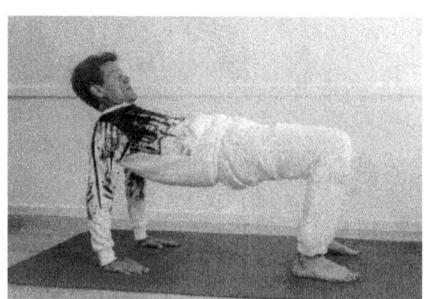

Step Three: Moving Securely to the Horizontal Position

Steps one and two gave you the opportunity to build up enough muscular force for this Tibetan exercise. In step three we will now get you gradually used to the horizontal position. Rest a few moments in this position. You need to decide whether to breathe in or out when being horizontal. One must definitely not stop the flow of breathing. Do not hold your breath while in the table position. Lots of beginners make exactly this exact mistake. Please consciously and slowly get used to the neck taking part in this horizontal position because you are then looking up to the ceiling. Then, while in the horizontal position, tense all your muscles including your facial musculature. This is quite a difficult and strenuous part of the fourth rite. It is not easy. Tense your muscles for a short period of max. 4 seconds.

Step Four: Breathing Correctly while Tensing Your Muscles

On principle, there are two alternatives to breathing while tensing one's muscles in the horizontal position. Either one can continue to inhale, or change over to exhaling during the 4-5 seconds of tensing the muscles. If you opt for inhaling while tensing the muscles, you will switch to breathing out and then gently lower your body back to the ground. In the second alternative, the inhaling -phase is short and quite forceful so that you can begin to exhale in the horizontal position. Breathing out is usually quite a bit longer, which is an argument for the second alternative. Every single practitioner should try it out for themselves and find what's best for them.

Step Five: Building Up One's Muscles

The tensing of the muscles makes the fourth Tibetan exercise very difficult. Therefore, I would like to suggest at this point a pre-exercise to build up enough muscle power to successfully carry it out. Lie down on the back and relax. Breathe in and out deeply and evenly. Now, tense all of your muscles. This is an important part of the fourth rite. Hence, we train it separately in this step number five. Quite a few people actually forget about this part altogether. Tense all muscles including your facial muscles. I am aware that especially women generally do not like "pull faces" or tense muscles in their faces. It is probably a beauty thing. I still want to suggest doing it and this is the reason why: even a very brief tensing of muscles helps open up the blood vessels, especially when being followed by relaxation. Therefore, it is safe to assume that flexing and tensing our muscles actually serves our health; moreover, it brings about a healthy facial colour.

Step Six: The Complete Fourth Tibetan

You have now done all the individual parts of this fourth exercise. You have gotten to know your own musculature pretty well. Moreover, you have made up your mind with the help of step three about whether or not to keep on inhaling when tensing your muscles in the horizontal position. Now it's time to tackle this exercise in its entirety.

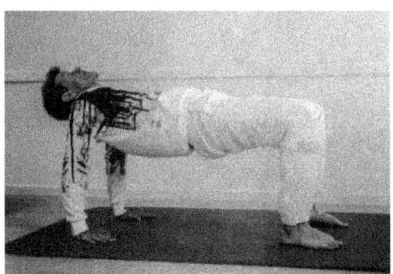

Start from the initial relaxed position lying on the floor. Now begin to inhale and push your entire body up. Please support this with your hands and feet resting all solidly on the ground. Push until you have fully reached the horizontal position. There, tense all your muscles for a few moments. Then relax your muscles again, and while exhaling gently move your entire body back to the ground. Then, relax fully for at least one full breath.

Rejoice, and be proud of yourself because you really have achieved something great. This exercise is far from being easy, and on the contrary, it's quite demanding. This is the case not only for an elderly, ill, or recovering person, but also by general standards. In addition, most of us ain't twenty no more!

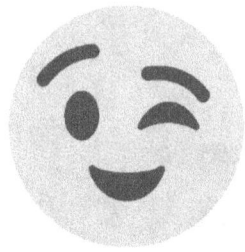

Common Errors and Corrections for the Fourth Tibetan

- It is very common that people do the pushing -up of their bodies too abruptly. Eventually, I figured out that this is because people either still feel insecure about the movement, or else they are not yet physically strong enough to push themselves up evenly and gently. Then, in order to "get through the exercise at all" they hasten through it. Even though that's completely understandable, it still takes a cut out of the health-benefits because a good muscle tone not only is attractive, but it protects your vital organs from most damage. Ultimately, you need to push up your body with your own strength. Therefore, I recommend that you first build up the required muscle force by exercising steps one, two, and four. As soon as your musculature meets with the required strength and you and your body have become conscious of this (new) fact, you will be able to carry out the upwards movement sufficiently gently and smoothly. As a matter of fact, both the upwards and the downward movements are meant to be gentle. In addition, you can support both by breathing evenly throughout the exercise.

- The next common mistake is to intersperse interruptions or even breaks during the upward- or the downward- movements. Yet, not even the short horizontal

position is actually a "stop". The reason being that tra-
ditionally, we qualify the tensing of the muscles as a
continuation of moving. This tensing of the muscles is
similar to the famous Qi -Gong exercise "Transform
into a mountain" (cf. Tippach "Opening the 9 Gates").
There, too, the stance is the Yin- or quiet/resting
phase, whereas the tensing of the muscles constitutes
the Yang- or moving phase.

- Another mistake is to push up your body too high, especially the hips. It is correct to bring yourself into a
horizontal position, but not further up, neither with the
head nor the hips. Thus, your entire body above the
knees forms a straight line.

- A closely connected mistake is bending the neck too
far back so that the top of your head actually points at
the ground. I do believe that this comes from being
overly motivated. Such additional bending of the neck
would be misplaced here. He or she who can really
bend their neck that far backwards has the opportunity to apply these skills in the Third Tibetan exercise. I would also like to point to the danger of injuring
oneself with such acrobatic moves. All of the above
can only be safely recommended to very advanced
students and real practitioners.

- Furthermore, some practitioners (mostly females) often forget to tense their musculature fully and in particular their facial muscles. It is correct to tense all of

one's muscles (from head to toe) for a short time only, but really hard.

- A common mistake is to stop breathing while tensing the muscles. Please keep your breath steady the whole time. Inhale and exhale evenly and without any inter-ruptions. Remember that harmonizing one's breathing with one's movements is also a mental achievement. If you want, read step four once more. If you prefer, you may transition from inhaling to exhaling *during* the phase of tensing your muscles. This is actually very good, but it is also quite difficult.

The Fifth Tibetan: The Reversed "V"

The Fifth Tibetan rite stands out because it is relatively easy to perform. Moreover, and probably more importantly, there is hardly anybody who would not agree that this exercise simply creates joy and a good mood in whoever practices it. Coming from more than a quarter of a century of experience, I can assure you that everybody to whom I taught this Tibetan will unanimously confirm that practically everyone feels vitalized, refreshed and full of inner joy after doing this rite. The core idea of the Fifth rite is to gently stretch the spine with an upward followed by a downward movement. During this stretch of the spine, one can also wonderfully fill one's lungs with plenty of air and oxygen.

At the same time, we have here an exercise which strengthens the spine and lungs enormously. This Tibetan is surely an exercise that contributes vastly to your overall health by general standards. The reason being that the fifth strengthens your entire musculature as well as heart and respiratory system. Moreover, it helps in becoming and maintaining flexibility. Even the anatomical term for it is simple: in colloquial terms it is the "reversed V". I am always looking forward to this one whether practicing for myself or teaching. This one is real fun. I hope that you are going to enjoy it just as much!

Before we start, I'd like to give one more piece of advice to all of you. It is probably best to perform this exercise barefoot. It is generally ok to use shoes or socks with studs, but for this exercise, one really needs to stand firmly on the ground. I had quite a few people in my workshops who take off their shoes and socks for this final fifth exercise, even though they generally do the other Tibetans with their shoes on.

You start by lying flat on your stomach breathing in. Put your hands on the ground close to your shoulders. Many of you may know a similar hand position from the Yoga -exercise "cobra". Your heels are up, the foot is resting on the toes, and your feet point upwards at a 90° angle. This Tibetan consists of bringing your body from this position (photo below on the left) up to your target -position (photo on the right) and back. Your breathing should be deep, and supported by your dia-phragm.

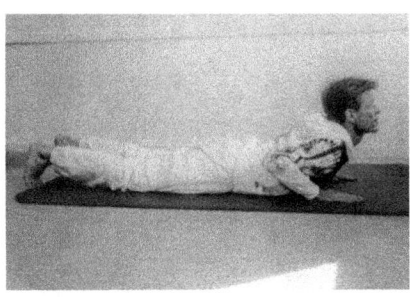

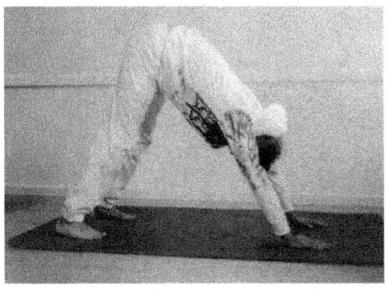

We can see here very well, how all Tibetan exercises work nicely together to give our bodies a complete and unified force (Prana); simply compare the different breathing rhythms in the third and the fifth exercises! Some parts energize us, others help us relax. In the third Tibetan the inhaling -phase happens while we bend our neck backwards. By contrast, in the fifth Tibetan we breathe in while bringing our chin towards our chest while bending our neck forwards.

Breathe in fully while lying on your stomach, then, begin exhaling. During the exhaling-phase gently lift your neck and bend in slightly backwards. At the same time, push your upper body upwards by the force of your arms and hands. Do not straighten your elbows fully but allow them to carry your body weight and build up some tension in your upper body and arms. This way you are going to reach the "V"-position.

Continue now with the second part of the movement breathing in! Push your buttocks up and straighten your legs. Here, it is important to straighten your arms too so that they can support your body well. Moreover, with the first repetition, move your feet a little more to your hands. That needs to happen because otherwise one cannot get one's buttocks up enough. The overall result and the target position of this exercise is a reversed "V". While moving upwards, inhale.

There is some discussion amongst those who practice the Tibetan exercises regularly, namely about the position of the heels in the V -position. Some say that the heels should touch the ground, others contend the exact opposite. Personally, I want to teach based on clear and plausible criteria. Now, since I am pretty lithe and well trained, but can still not extend my ligaments enough to fully put my heels down in this position (cf. photo above on the right), I do not want to expect anything from anyone that I cannot properly perform myself. Hence, each one of you needs to establish for themselves what works best for you. Personally, I think that it actually makes no difference at all whether or not your heels touch the floor in the reversed V-position.

Simplified Version of the Fifth Tibetan

Every reader may establish for themselves how easy (or not so easy) this exercise is for them. Quite often though, the pushing up of the buttocks into the position of the "reversed V" is seen as difficult. For this reason, I have developed along with many older participants in my workshops a version which is a lot easier. For this, you probably need another blanket or cushion for under your knees. The simplification consists in not bringing up your buttocks with one push, but first bringing yourself onto your knees, for which you need the additional blanket (cf. photo below).

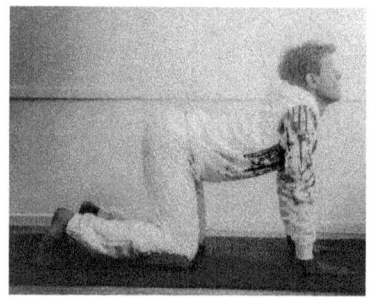

Once up on your knees, breathe in and out again. During the next inhaling phase, push up from the in-between- position to the V -position. You will surely find this a lot easier to do. Over time, your musculature in your arms and legs will get stronger, and eventually strong enough for you to be able to perform the original version of the Fifth Tibetan. Even if that should not be the case, please rest assured that you will still be able to do the lighter version at the age of 100.

Respect your body and thank it for having carried you through your entire life. Give it the rest that it needs, and that it de-serves.

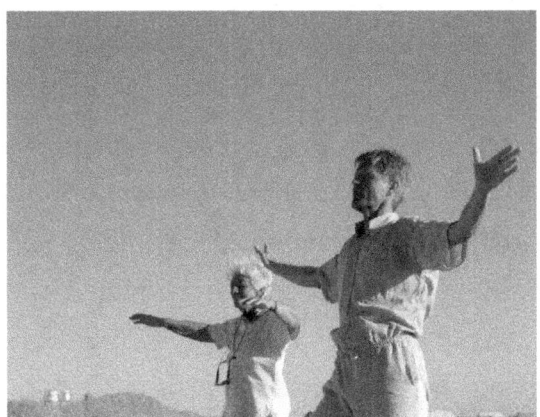

Common Errors and Corrections for the Fifth Tibetan

- Quite often people mix up their breathing patterns, namely they breathe in during the downward movement. My guess is that they are used to one overall breathing principle, which is to breathe out during the strenuous part of an exercise. Since pushing up and getting into the V -position is somewhat more strenuous than the rest of the fifth rite, some just try to coordinate that part with their breathing out. One may argue that pushing oneself up with one's elbows and bending one's neck backwards is even more strenuous. Be that as it may, we do have to consider that breathing in while bending the neck backwards is already prevalent in exercise three. Therefore, the correct breathing pattern is inhaling while getting into the V - position.

- The second most common error which I have observed many times is that people forget to bend their neck forward (the chin-towards-chest -movement) while pushing up into the V. Quite obviously this exercise wants us to bend our spine as much as possible. This includes our neck. Hence, the only correct way of doing this is to also bend our neck, which includes moving your chin towards our chest when pushing upwards. This then fully vitalizes the spine and thus our energy vortices and chakras. Moreover, the exercises before this one have helped us a good deal to strengthen our neck muscles. It therefore makes perfect sense for us to now include the neck in our bending of the spine in order to include our heads as well. Bending the neck opens this joint very efficiently and allows positive vibrations and the life force Qi that in turn contributes vastly to the joyful sensations brought about by doing this particular exercise. In addition, bending our neck is excellent for our throat chakra and thus promotes healthy thyroid glands. The latter helps regulate our hormonal wellbeing as well as our entire endocrine system. Both movements of the neck need to be well controlled and relatively slow. Please never throw your neck around wildly or in an uncontrolled fashion.

- The same kind of mistake would be to inhale while bending the neck backwards. Begin the fifth exercise in a quiet and lying position breathing out. Breathe in, then breathe out again beginning the active part of this exercise by pushing your upper body onto your elbows and bending your neck backwards. Then, inhaling, you straighten your elbows while pushing your buttocks up into the V. This way you make sure that your breathing pattern always remains correct, thus supporting your overall health quite considerably.

- Sometimes, people forget to tense their buttock muscles while pushing up into the V. In addition, quite often, people forget to relax these muscles when lowering the buttocks again. It is beneficial to tense your buttock muscles very firmly. People often talk of exercising to strengthen "stomach, legs, and buttocks" and this exercise superbly supports your efforts in this direction. Moreover, tensing and relaxing one's buttock muscles helps to de-stress your entire lower back which prevents back pains from occurring.

The True Sixth Tibetan

Since the early 80s, various teachers have taught a breathing exercise combined with a bending of the upper body and resting one's hands on the knees as the Sixth Tibetan. This is not a bad exercise as we know from both Qi -Gong and Yoga, this is merely a preparatory exercise helping to loosen up and harmonizing one's breathing. In truth though, this is not a Tibetan rite, despite Peter Kelder depicting it in his book.

The real thing is that we can combine each of the Five Tibetans with a mantra. In. In this way our mental, emotional, and spiritual development can keep up with our physical strengthening. Ultimately, we do not only be or experience ourselves as a body. Rather, we want to fully become conscious of our own spirituality because real health comprises a lot more than physical aspects, namely just as much an inner mindfulness and the ability to get into a state of being connected. That's why I would like to recommend you try the following mantra:

"I Am One with the Great Spirit"

In order for you to get used to the inner repetition of such a mantra, it is advisable to recite it first in a lying position right before and right after an exercise.

Or you can first speak your mantra internally after each individual exercise during the transition phases while breathing evenly. Before and after training the Five Tibetans you may like to use the following mantra:

"The Spirit in Me
Greets the Spirit in You"

I would like to recommend for you all to choose such a mantra according to your individual needs and preferences. It needs to be in harmony with your current wishes and positive thoughts in a wholesome way. Therefore, there cannot be a wrong or a right mantra, wording, or affirmation that comes from a manual. We are all different and we change over time.

In general, I find it to be a mistake to add this dimension based on intentions and wants which stem from our minds. The Tibetans encompass some wonderful spiritual gymnastics, which we should keep free from our small egos. Instead, we should aim at not using them for a specific mind-driven goal. In case you find such mantras or affirmations silly, you simply do not relate to them, or it hinders you from properly concentrating on the exercises, simply leave them out. Not adding them will in no way affect your health negatively or take away from the beauty and majestic that lies in their movements.

The "In-Between -Phases" or Transitions

Concluding this book, I would like to describe in some detail these very important phases between the individual rites. Generally speaking, these phases serve your relaxation and harmonization. They are a lot more than simply pauses or rests. "Exercising" (i.e. "*gong*"), means producing Yang -energies. Resting creates more Yin in us. In order for these two forces or polarities to harmonize well with one another, the phases in between the exercises needs to be quiet and serene. You need to support it with regular harmonizing breathing. An additional and helpful mantra could be:

"I Am One with My Breath"
(or) "I Am My Breathing"

Please consider these phases more than just resting, non-existing, or pausing. Rather, live them as an expression of and an opportunity to unite all forces within you and form a togetherness. It helps to move very slowly, carefully, and quietly. Abstain from any hectic or abrupt movement. This way, all the rites become one within you and with you.

If necessary, please simply insert extra pauses between repetitions or the individual rites. Sit on the ground or on the earth, on your mat, or on a chair. Alternatively, simply lie down. Wait until you feel rested and revitalized. Come back into your equilibrium. Do not allow your sports ambitions to take over. He or she who needs a very long pause between exercises, has most likely applied too much force and strain during the exercise itself. In that case, it is certainly better to reduce the force put in until they can do with a smaller pause to get back into their equilibrium.

Indulge in a sip of tea or enjoy some fresh water in between exercises if you like.

However, do not eat.

Any form of activity would be wrong.

Please be focused and stay concentrated! Think lovingly of your body, your sensations, and perceptions. Do not do or think of anything other than that, namely do not use your phone no matter how short the conversation. No checking of messages or Facebook. Once more, I'd like to point out to the care and mindfulness which late -comers, elderly, or ill persons should apply at the junctures between the exercises. The reason being that this way your mind and body get a realistic chance to absorb positive vital energies and convert them into long-lasting health.

Take this time and use it to harmonize all parts of you with your own self and your breathing. Allow your movements to flow evenly.

The Transition Phase after the First Tibetan Rite

Allow me to expand a little more on the transition phase after the first rite. The photos below show some positions which are useful between the first and the second rite in order to deepen and intensify the health benefits. My wish to all of you, from the bottom of my heart, is that you may soon sense and perceive how the energy keeps on gently spinning in your back and/or your entire body, once you stop spinning around and hold your basic stance.

In Qi -Gong, we call this phenomenon "feel the Yang within the Yin" and it is considered as one of the ten jewels of eternal life. The photo below on the right-hand side shows another good base stance with "empty" fists, which means "without any tension in arms or hands". This stance is widespread in Qi -Gong as well as in advanced forms of Tai Chi, and we do consider it very relaxing.

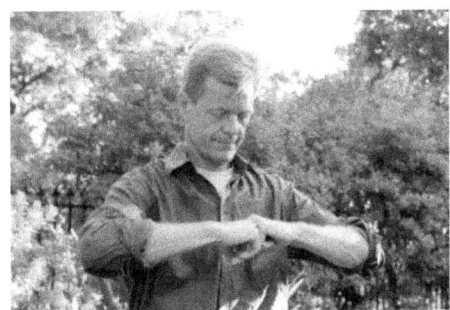

The transition -phases can be of varying lengths. Should you feel dizzy or even nauseous, you really need to remain quiet until that passes. This may take longer today than it did yesterday. Sit down if necessary. It would be so wrong to put any additional strain on yourself. Rather, remain in the relaxing base stance standing - quite similar to the base stance in Qi –Gong - which is a mixture of standing and sitting. Hold your arms loose and do not flex any muscles. Depending on which relaxing stance you choose for yourself, you could go into a quiet and meditative inner space. Younger or quite dynamic people, who still want too much, often do this wrong.

Transition Phase after the Second Tibetan Exercise

The second exercise is the one in which our feet point upwards at the beginning, then the legs are moved upwards and gently brought back on the ground while exhaling. This rite is pretty demanding, especially for beginners, which is why we have looked at it in detail and listed individual steps hereinbefore. Now, we should adapt each transition phase to the exercise before it. Hence, the high degree of strain caused by the second rite will potentially require a longer relaxing - phase.

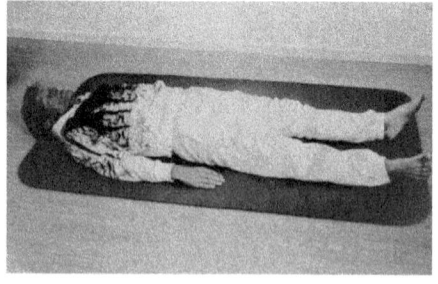

Since lying down is even more relaxing than standing quietly, it is probably best to remain lying down after the final repetition. Stretch yourself out on the ground and breathe evenly in and out. With our breathing, we do actually manage our relaxation phase. The more deeply and evenly we can breathe, the more quickly we regain our composure and inner harmony. Breathing correctly can be wonderfully calming for our mind and body. If you prefer it, you may close your eyes here. Remain lying on the ground for up to 4 minutes.

Every person perceives certain physical positions as more or less relaxing. However much some amongst us may think that it is the most relaxing thing to just lie on your back - this can be quite different in others. Quite a few of the participants in my courses, and in particular the elderly people, find it relaxes them even better to put at least one of their knees up at an angle or lean it onto the other knee (cf. photo below).

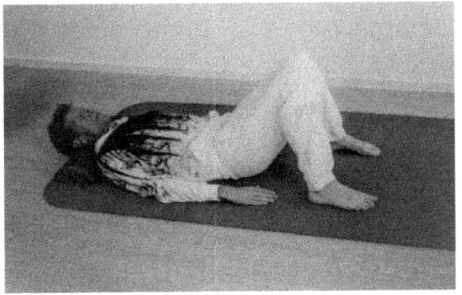

Surely, an argument in favour of this position is that our sinews is less stretched out than when both legs are lying directly on the ground next to one another. One woman suggested, quite rightly in my eyes, to lean one knee to the side and prop it up with a sufficiently hard cushion. Please try this out for yourself, because you need to feel this personally, rather than copying the "correct" position from a book.

The Transition -Phase after the Third Tibetan Rite

In the third exercise we very gently bent our spine, back, and necks backwards. This requires us to make sure that, during this transition phase, we afford the maximum possible relaxation to our back, and especially to our lower back. There are several solutions on offer, and every one of you will probably find them to be more or less relaxing for your backs. Simply choose your very own position that feels good for yourself.

Whatever relaxes you most is currently the best alternative for you. The most advanced position that I have seen at this juncture is the leaf-position, which you may know from practicing classical Hatha Yoga (c.f. photo below). Most people in my classes have found this leaf -Asana (that's the term for this "position" which we use in yoga) too difficult if not outright undoable, or not relaxing. Since I do not intend to teach yoga in this book, I shall limit it to the photo below. He or she who can do it, will probably find it far more relaxing than it may look at first sight.

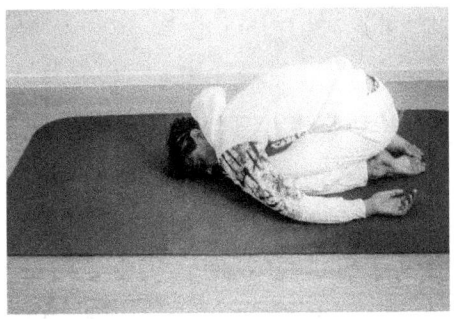

For someone who is (still) a little less lithe, the following positions may prove helpful and relaxing here as well:

- Simply sitting with legs at an angle or legs pointing outward to the sides (cf. photo below)

- Sitting in tailor position with your hands resting behind your back (cf. photo below on the right)

I am sure that everyone who practices regularly will make the right choice for themselves. Please remember that you want to stretch your back here, or at least you support it well.

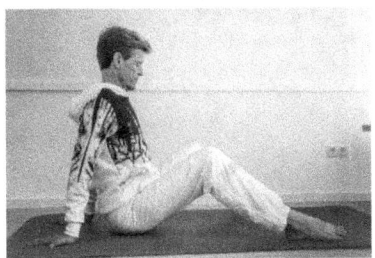 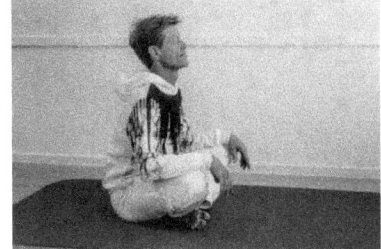

Most people find it very relaxing to sit on their calves. The good thing about this position in particular is that you simply have to lower your body after doing this exercise in order to get there (cf. photo down below on the left). In this position, your buttocks rest on your calves, and your feet are moved from the 90 -degree angle during the exercise so that the back of your feet rest on the ground. He or she who meditates every now and then knows that one can remain in this position quite comfortably and in a relaxed fashion for quite some time. Should you want to meditate a little at this juncture, simply sit on your calves, and put your hands with palms facing up in your laps Close your eyes and start to sense and feel how relaxation and feelings of heavy and quiet start almost immediately to circulate pleasantly within you (cf. photo below on the right).

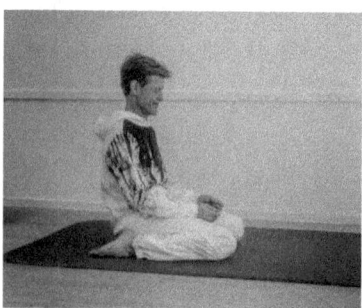 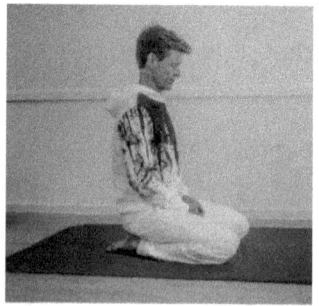

However, quite a few people reported experiencing foot pain in this position. Since we have agreed to make sure not to incur pains during the exercises, the same holds true for the transition phase between the exercises. Please try this out and establish for yourselves which position is best for you.

Transition -Phase after the Fourth Tibetan Rite

The fourth exercise was the one in which we bring ourselves to a horizontal position, and then while exhaling we lowered ourselves gently back to a seated starting position. Personally, I think this one is the most challenging Tibetan exercise. Since this one is definitely demanding in a physical sense as well, we have to make sure that the resting or transitory position is one in which we can truly gather our forces.

Relax.

Breathe!

In.

And out again.

There are several possible resting positions:

- Sitting in what can be called the "Lotus"- position

- Sitting with one leg crossed over the other leg

- Simple sitting position with half-stretched legs

- If it feels right and relaxing to you, it is a good idea to allow your neck and upper body to let go. Lower your chin to your chest and let it rest there

- Sitting on your calves as shown in the paragraph above

- Sitting with your knees at a comfortable angle, with both your upper body and your neck resting on the knees

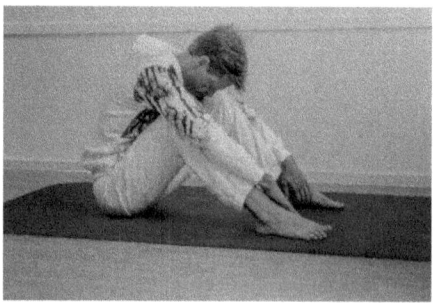

Final Resting -Phase

Usually your training session ends after the fifth exercise. Simply lie down on your stomach, if it is comfortable enough, and rest. Put your hands on either side of your body. Feel one with yourself! Breathe deeply and evenly. Quietly be aware of your body, and of how you have been giving something wonderful to yourself. If you so wish, stay in this position for some time.

Personally, I find it very important not to jump up right after the physical training, when having concluded your Tibetan exercises. Do not rush back to "doing –mode" immediately. The fifth exercise can be especially vitalizing. I do suggest you allow your body enough time to absorb the positive effects. It is one of the greatest mistakes of the Western mind that we all want to *do* something with the fresh energy which we have generated.

Our life energy, the "Qi", should ideally not be consumed by our next activity. Rather, the Qi should have time and space to support our self-healing forces and to slow down our aging process or even reverse it. Hence my whole-hearted suggestion that you take at least 15 minutes to rest. Concluding now, let us have a closer look at suitable postures to do that. Every reader can of course make their own choices according to their needs and personal comfort.

Remaining on your stomach is the first possibility. Many people like it and can simply rest on their mats. Others prefer putting a cushion under their heads. Depending on the out-side temperature, one should put a blanket on because it is vital that your body stays warm. You may want to sleep for a bit. Maybe think of your favourite mantra and slumber away over it.

Alternatively, you may choose from the following relaxing positions:

- Lie on your back and put a blanket over your body to keep yourself warm

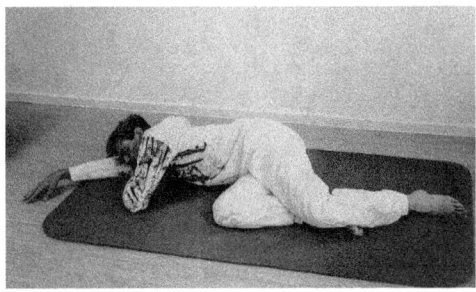

- Lie on your stomach and gently roll up your body to get into what we call the fetal position

- Use a sleeping position with one of your legs tilted up about halfway. Actually, this position seems to be relaxing and comfortable for most people. Relax your neck and allow your head to roll gently to the side

- Use parts of any of the aforementioned suggestions and combine them in your very own and personal way

Sleep well, or just relax.

Allow your body to absorb the forces you gained. The resting –position after the Fifth is also the concluding position for your training today. Once you get here, you will probably en-joy a relaxed, meditative state of mind.

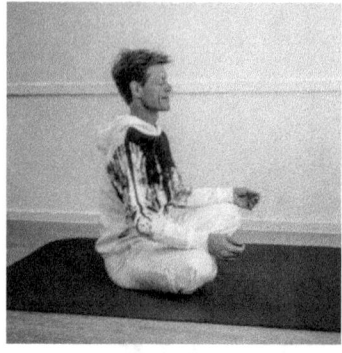 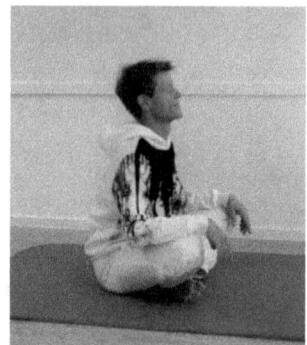

Congratulations!

And thank you for your trust!

I wish you the very best!

Stay healthy and enjoy life.

Remain strong!

Dr. Stefan Ulrich Tippach Ph.D.